figure it out

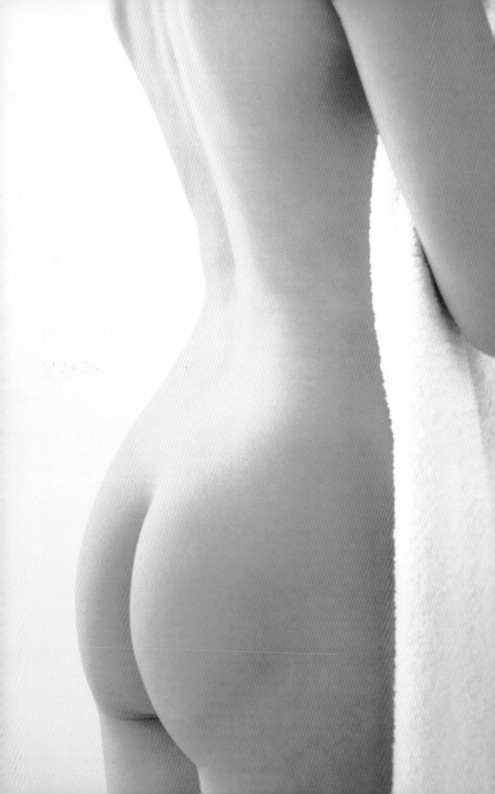

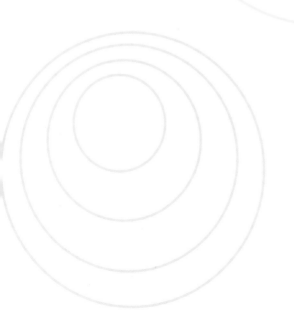

Wendy Lewis

figure it out

the lowdown on reshaping your body

QUADRILLE

Editorial Director: Jane O'Shea

Creative Director: Mary Evans

Designer: Sue Storey

Project Editor: Lisa Pendreigh

Editor: Katie Ginn

Picture Research: Nadine Bazar

Illustrations: Sue Storey

Production: Nancy Roberts

First published in 2002 by Quadrille Publishing Limited
Alhambra House
27–31 Charing Cross Road
London WC2H OLS

Before following any advice or practice suggested in this book, it is recommended that you consult your doctor as to its suitability, especially if you suffer from any health problems or special conditions. The publishers, the author and the photographers cannot accept responsibility for any injuries or damage incurred as a result of following the exercises in this book or of using any of the therapeutic methods described or mentioned here.

Cataloguing-in-Publication Data: a catalogue record for this book is available from the British Library.

ISBN 1 903845 68 8

Printed and bound in Singapore

Contents

A gorgeous body takes a combination of good genes, healthy and active lifestyle, sensible diet and hard work. Nothing gives a woman a burst of self-confidence like knowing she's in good shape. It translates to the way she carries herself and how she fits into her clothes. Getting the body of your dreams may not always be possible, but getting a better one definitely is. Women crave information on the latest and greatest cellulite remedies, slimming techniques, fitness breakthroughs and body contouring treatments. Now girls can get the real scoop on an age-old quintessential beauty challenge – keeping their figure. This comprehensive guide delivers fresh solutions to the dilemma of dimples, bulges, how to jumpstart a fitness plan and decreasing your size – from prevention, to maintenance and ultimately, to correction. It features the lowdown on state-of-the-art methods, what works and what's a waste of money, top clinical advances, new para-surgical treatments, DIY home remedies, as well as resources for how to find a good doctor, shopping guides and web links.

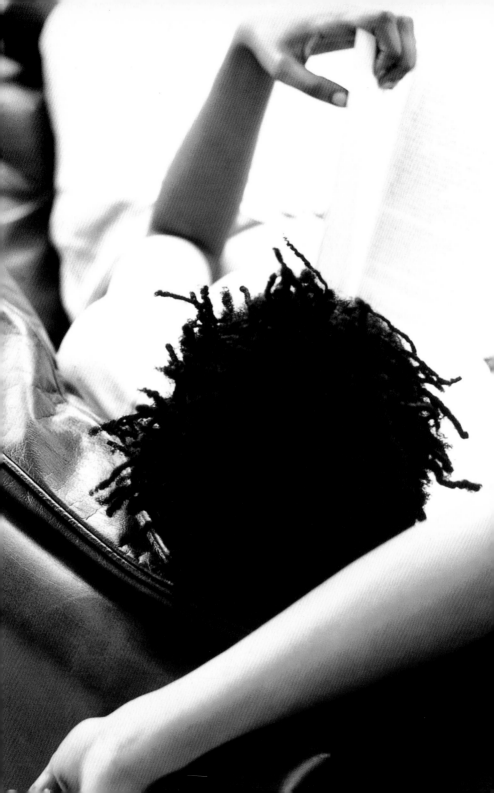

THE BASICS

THE BASICS

For centuries, women have been at war with their fat cells.
Doctors estimate that around half the population is heavier than
they should be, and about one quarter are at least 2 stone
overweight. Clearly, we're eating too much and moving too little.
Many of us sit in front of computers all day, then go home and
surf the net some more or sit in front of the TV until bedtime.
In spite of the constant bombardment of signals to eat less food
and more healthily and to exercise, many women are gaining weight
faster and are getting heavier by the day. Studies show that
being overweight increases your risk of dying young by at least
half, and you are more likely to have high blood pressure, high
cholesterol, diabetes, asthma, arthritis and some cancers,
including breast and colon cancer.

Losing weight isn't that hard; the difficult part is keeping
it off. All too often, our idea of a shape-up programme consists
of jumping on the latest fad diet bandwagon, which we inevitably
fall off when we get bored with it or it stops working. Plan on
losing weight slowly and forget about looking for quick fixes.
The ultimate measure of your success is your bodyfat percentage.

fat stats

Women have a basic love / hate relationship with fat. We are one eighth more likely to be obese than men and 99 per cent of us are desperate to avoid becoming fat.

This sentiment accounts for the proliferation of diets, miracle pills, power drinks and gym memberships. This three-letter word alone is enough to instill fear in the hearts of every woman with visions of lumps, bumps, bulges and saddlebags. On any given date, between 15 and 35 per cent of adults are dieting. 90 per cent of people with eating disorders are adolescents and young women. Fashion models weigh about one-quarter less than the average female. We live in a culture in which fatness is considered tantamount to failure, and the pressure to be thin is very real to most women. Size still matters when it comes to determining self-worth or attractiveness. A woman's dress size has become inextricably linked with her identity. There are some women who don't store fat and can consume twice as many calories as the rest of us without gaining an ounce. No one said life is fair. The good news is that most women aren't as fat as they think they are.

Women struggle to control their fat, and will go to great lengths to lose it to the point of starvation. Everyone knows that the safest way to lose weight is to eat a nutritionally complete diet, low in calories and fat. Burning off more calories than you take in will cause you to lose weight. If you lose the weight slowly, you'll be much more effective at keeping it off, especially if you incorporate exercise into your routine. Excess fat can be reduced by limiting caloric intake to a level below the energy exerted, or increasing physical activity. The bad news is that there is no magic formula, and there is no one diet or plan that works for everyone. The typical unhealthy diet is loaded with sugar and fats, but contains less than the recommended amounts of fruits and vegetables. Every diet seems to have one common underlying theme – French fries and Sara Lee are out.

Generally, an older body is a fatter body. An average 20-year-old woman's body is $16^1/_2$ per cent muscle, 47 per cent non-muscle lean tissue, 10 per cent bone and $26^1/_2$ per cent fat. By comparison, the average 20-something guy has 30 per cent muscle and only 18 per cent fat. The differences between women and men increase with age. Both sexes become fatter, but women become more so. Excess fat settles in different places at different stages of life. The major culprit is oestrogen.

Teens and 20s – Any excess fat is distributed evenly around your body.
30s and 40s – Extra weight goes straight to your hips and thighs.
50s – Added pounds head for your waistline and stay put.
60s and 70s – If you have been steadily gaining weight through the years, expect to be somewhat pear-shaped.

The older you get, the harder it is to lose weight because your body settles in, gets lazy and grows accustomed to your fat. The shifting also tends to follow the pattern of gravity – it gets lower. In general, there is a tendency for the shoulders to narrow, the chest size to grow and the pelvis to widen over the years. Chest size in women peaks between the ages of 55 and 64. Although a bigger chest may seem like something to look forward to, it is usually accompanied by the flattening and sagging of the breasts. After age 65, a woman's chest generally shrinks. The pelvis, in contrast, keeps widening throughout life, which accounts for the pear shape period.

body mass

Body weight represents a sum of the bodily structures including muscle and bone, body water and stored fat. One measure of plumpness is the dreaded Body Mass Index (BMI), which at first glance, reads like an Einstein theory in physics.

BMI is determined by dividing your weight in pounds by your height in inches squared, and then multiplying by 705. For example, a woman who is 5'6" and weighs 13½ stone would have a BMI of 31, as follows:

You are considered overweight if your BMI is 25–29.9. Obesity kicks in if you have a BMI of 30 or higher. However, not every woman fits neatly into BMI charts or height / weight statistics. If you have a large amount of muscle, which weighs more than fat, for example, your weight may seem higher than normal limits. Lean body mass is commonly used to describe the muscles in your arms, legs, back, neck and abdomen. Another measure doctors use is your body composition, which is your proportion of fat to muscle. A woman needs to have a minimum of 13–17 per cent body fat for regular menstruation. If it is lower than that, periods may stop and you could become infertile. Menstrual cycle irregularities may also compromise healthy bones. The healthy ranges of body fat are significantly higher for women than for men, and the

BMI

165 cm = 1.65 m

1.65 squared = 2.7225

60 kg divided by 2.7225 = 22.04

Age	Healthy range of body fat
18–39	21–32%
40–59	23–33%
60–79	24–35%

range increases slightly with age. For women, if your body fat is greater than 27–30 per cent, you would be considered overweight.

Not all fat is created equal

We all need some fat. It is vital for the maintenance of healthy skin and hair. Although everyone has a smooth layer of fat, individual amounts depend on weight, lifestyle and genetics. This fat layer is an insulator for the body and cushions the organs, muscles and nerves to protect them from injury. Cellulite, on the other hand, is lumpy and provides no padding whatsoever. Then there is the visceral fat that can collect around the mid-section and surround the organs. This can present the greatest risk to your health. Lipids seep into the bloodstream from this layer and can cause high cholesterol and cardiovascular disease.

Fat substitute

In 1996, Olestra, made with soyabean or cottonseed oil, was approved by the US Food and Drug Administration (FDA) for use in snacks such as crisps, chips and crackers. Its chemical composition adds no fat or calories. A 30 g serving of crisps fried with Olestra contains 75 calories and no fat, as opposed to regular crisps, which have 150 calories and 10 fat grams per ounce. Olestra may cause abdominal cramping and loose stools, and may inhibit the absorption of some nutrients like vitamins A, D, E and K.

fat facts

*Fat is essential for the body to function properly. It is vital –
the most concentrated source of energy in foods.*

Essential fat – found in small amounts in your bone marrow, organs,
central nervous system and muscles.

Storage fat – accumulated primarily beneath the skin but is also found in
other areas in the body.

False fat – some excess weight is 'false fat' or the excess bloat that comes
from hypersensitivity to many common foods. We feel and look a lot better
without it. It also comes off fastest. The loss of false fat is one of the
reasons people sometimes lose weight quickly at the beginning of a new diet.

Fats are high in calories. Diets with less than 20 per cent fat can leave you
unsatisfied and more likely to overeat when your willpower crumbles. Fat
stimulates the release of a hormone that slows the rate of food leaving the

BEAUTY BYTE:

Want to learn more about body fat analysis? Log on to
www.fatcheck.com or www.feelingfat.net.

stomach. The stomach and intestine are lined with receptors that, when
stimulated by fat, signal the brain that you're full. After the first 20 minutes of
exercise when the body has used up the calories from carbs, it begins to
depend on those from fat.

Your fat IQ

True or false? There is a healthy range of body fat and it is the same for men and women.
False. For the average adult, the healthy range of body fat for women is 21–35 per cent; for men it is 8–24 per cent.

True or false? The more lean body mass (muscle) you have, the easier it is to maintain your weight.
True. It is easier to maintain your weight if you have a greater amount of lean body mass, because it results in a higher metabolic rate. Therefore, you burn more calories when you are sitting or lying down.

True or false? Strength or resistance training can help you increase your lean body mass.
True. Lean body mass can be increased by a combination of strength and resistance training.

True or false? When you lose weight, you only lose fat.
False. When you lose weight, you lose both lean mass and fat. To maintain your metabolic rate and stay healthy, it's better to preserve lean body mass and muscles as much as possible and reduce your body fat.

True or false? To lose weight, it doesn't matter what kind of method you use as long as your weight goes down.
False. When you lose weight, you want to reduce your body fat while preserving your lean body mass.

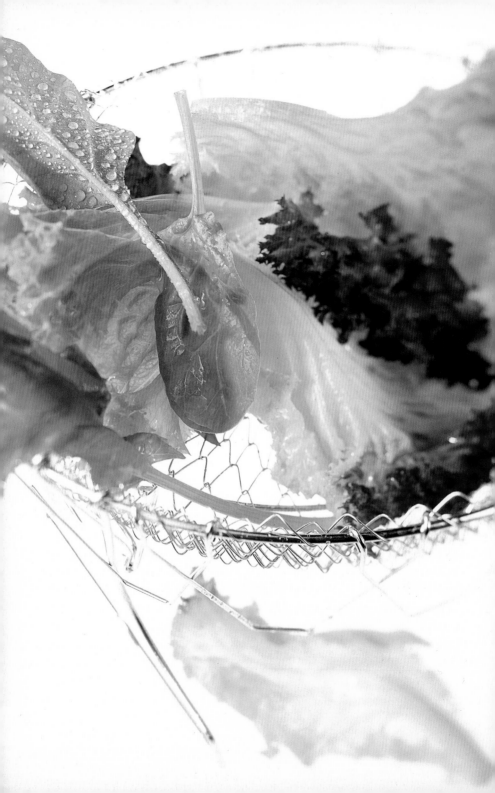

FAT FREEDOM

FAT FREEDOM

Fats are organic compounds made up of carbon, hydrogen and oxygen, which belong to a group of substances called lipids. Fat provides 9 calories per gram, more than twice the number provided by carbohydrates or protein. Fats provide the essential fatty acids, which are not made by the body and must be obtained from food. Fatty acids provide the raw materials that help in the control of blood pressure, blood clotting, inflammation and other bodily functions, and are the primary components of dietary fats. Omega-3 fatty acid or fish oil is a polyunsaturated fat found in seafood, particularly fatty fish like salmon. This is a type of fat that helps increase healthy cholesterol, decrease bad cholesterol in the blood, and may lower blood pressure by lowering triglycerides.

Fat helps in the absorption of the fat-soluble vitamins A, D and E, and to maintain the immune system. You don't want to eliminate it completely, just limit what you take in to what you need and nothing more. The key is to strike a healthy balance.

never say diet

In the last 20 years, the number of overweight women in their 20s has climbed by more than 60 per cent, and about half of all women in their 30s and 40s are considered overweight.

Few of us live our lives at our ideal weight on a daily basis. Diets offer only short term solutions; they are destined to become something you go on and come off because they are so limiting. The goal is to encourage long-term lifestyle change.

It is difficult to maintain dramatic, significant weight loss for long periods. Set realistic goals. Aim for something that you feel can be maintained for 6 months. If you overindulge one day, don't waste precious time and energy feeling guilty, but get back on track the next day. If you're not sure you're really hungry, wait 20 minutes before you eat and you may find you weren't that hungry at all. Never let yourself get too famished or you'll be tempted to eat whatever is within reach.

Losing even as little as 5–10 per cent of your body weight can make major health improvements. It helps glucose tolerance, blood pressure and blood lipids because they improve on a continuum of weight loss. The simplest method is to decrease intake by 250 calories a day and increase expenditure by the same amount. If you exercise following weight loss, you will be more successful in keeping the weight off. Exercise changes the body so that it can handle fat, by burning it as a primary fuel. It also revs up your metabolism and turns your body into a fat-burning machine.

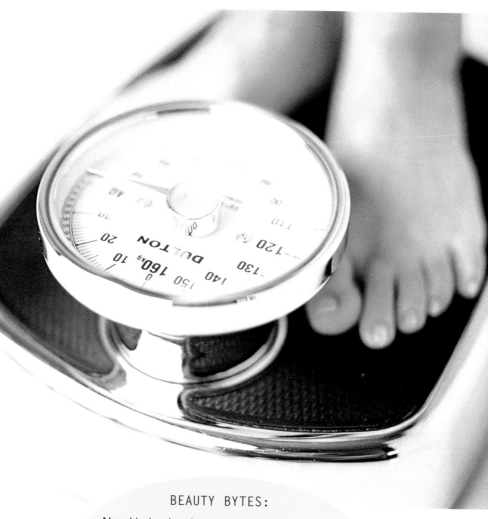

BEAUTY BYTES:

Need help planning a diet you can stick to?

Who doesn't? Log onto these sites:

www.ediets.com, www.cyberdiet.com,

www.mynutrition.co.uk and

www.nutrition.gov

just the fat

Counting fat grams is one way to get a clear picture of your daily totals. The trick is to maintain a diet of less than 30 per cent fat.

'I'm eating fat-free foods, so why aren't I losing weight?' 'I'm counting fat grams instead of calories, but I'm still fat!' If that sounds familiar, you're not alone. Don't assume that because a food is called fat-free, you can eat as much as you want. Nutritionists recommend reading labels and sticking to foods that have less than 5 fat grams. This allows you a treat of a few higher fat foods as long as they fit within your daily limit. If you only eat foods that are 30 per cent fat or lower, your diet is guaranteed to be less than 30 per cent fat, but that can be limiting. There will be times when you have a craving for something that measures higher than 30 per cent. Some fatty foods can be squeezed into a healthy diet if you only eat them occasionally, in moderation and as part of an otherwise low-fat diet. So you can nibble a couple of chocolate biscuits and still be okay, as long as you're not downing a pint of Häagen Dazs.

EXAMPLE

Total calories for day: 1950

Total fat grams: 36

36 fat grams x 9 calories per fat gram = 324 fat calories

Fat calories (324) divided by total calories (2069) = 16.6% of total calories are from fat

food diary

Sometimes putting it all on paper makes it official. At the end of the day, add up the fat grams and total calories. Work out your daily percentage by multiplying the fat grams by 9 to get fat calories. Divide this number by the total calories. The final number should be less than 30 per cent.

Day	Breakfast	Lunch	Dinner	Snacks	Calories	Fats
Monday						
Tuesday						
Wednesday						
Thursday						
Friday						
Saturday						
Sunday						

having a breakdown

The main function of carbohydrates is to provide energy to the brain and nervous system. The body breaks down starches and sugars into glucose, which it then uses for energy.

Complex carbohydrates are found in breads, cereals, legumes and rice. Simple carbohydrates naturally occur in fruits, vegetables and dairy products. They can also be found in processed and refined sugars. These only provide empty calories – lacking vitamins, minerals and fibre.

SUGAR
- Gets stored in the muscles
- Is burned first and most easily
- There is very little of it so it runs out quickly

FAT
- Gets stored far from the muscles
- Is harder to access when you start to exercise
- The supply is endless

The Good

Polyunsaturated fat – also known as essential fatty acids, these are highly unsaturated fats found in foods including corn, soya bean oil, salmon and mackerel. As the body can't manufacture these fats, it must get them from food.

Monounsaturated fat – found in large quantities in highly unsaturated fat, which is found in large amounts in foods from plants, including peanuts, avocados, olives and olive oil.

The bad

Saturated fat – causes cholesterol to build up in the arteries. Sources include meat, poultry, whole milk dairy products, chocolate, coconut and palm oil. Saturated fats tend to be solid at room temperature and raise blood cholesterol. Excessive consumption increases your risk of coronary heart disease and obesity. Saturated fat should be limited to 10 per cent of the total calories for the day. The remainder of the day's fat intake should be equal amounts of poly-unsaturated and monounsaturated fat.

Trans fat – manmade fats found in margarine, shortening, packaged baked goods, crackers and confectionary. The words 'hydrogenated' or 'partially hydrogenated' before any oil or fat are an indicator. They affect the body in a similar way to saturated fats.

fat busters

Given the advances in 'low' and 'non-fat' foods such as salad dressings and cakes, it seems only fair that the fat around our waists should shrink.

It is common to think that if food is low in fat, you can eat twice as much or as much as you want. Sadly, this is not the case. Stick to 'low-fat' and 'fat-free' products whenever possible, and be skeptical about labels and claims.

REALITY CHECK:
Alcohol can make you feel bloated and add on the pounds. For example, a 6oz glass of chardonnay contains 90 calories whilst half a pint of lager has 150 calories.

Don't forget to note the serving size used when looking at nutritional information on packets. If the serving size is 100 g, if you consume 200 g, remember that the amount of fat, sugar etc. doubles too.

Losing extra pounds involves more than counting calories and cutting back on fat. It's the little choices you make throughout the day that make or break your success. When it comes to weight loss, it's the number of calories that count, no matter what the source. The bottom line is: cut calories, increase exercise, lose weight.

Reading matters

What it says	What it means
Reduced fat	25% less fat than whatever it is being compared to
Light or lite	50% less fat than whatever it is being compared to
Low fat	One serving has fewer than 3 g of fat
Fat-free	One serving has less than 1/2 g of fat
Lean	Less than 10 g of fat, 4.5 g of saturated fat and 95 mg of cholesterol per serving and per 100 g (meats, seafood, poultry)
Extra lean	Less than 5 g of fat, 2 g of saturated fat and 95 mg of cholesterol per serving and 100 g
Cholesterol-free	Less than 2 mg cholesterol and 2 g or less saturated fat per serving
Low cholesterol	20 mg or less cholesterol per serving and 2 g or less saturated fat per serving
High fibre	5 g or more fibre per serving
Sugar-free	Less than 0.5 g of sugar per serving
Sodium-free	Less than 5 mg sodium per serving
Low sodium	140 mg or less per serving
Light (in sodium)	50% reduction in sodium

magic bullets

Diet supplements, fat burners and energizers come and go. Every few months another miracle pill hits the market. The purpose is always the same: a cure for fat without any effort.

Diet drugs can produce weight loss for a while, but as soon as you stop taking them, the weight comes right back on unless you have changed your evil ways in the process. Pills can't change the way your body handles fat, they can only make temporary adjustments.

Appetite suppressants

The medications most often used in the management of obesity are 'appetite suppressants'. Appetite suppressant medications promote weight loss by decreasing appetite or increasing the feeling of being full. They decrease appetite by increasing serotonin or catecholamine, two brain chemicals that affect mood and appetite. Some antidepressants have also been used as appetite suppressants. Generally these medications can lead to an average weight loss of from 5 pounds to 1 1/2 stone above what would be expected by dieting alone. They are not recommended for someone who is only mildly overweight or has less than a stone to lose. If your health is compromised because of your weight and rapid weight loss is needed, a physician may also recommend drug therapy. Every woman responds differently to appetite suppressant medications, and some experience more weight loss than others. Maximum weight loss usually

occurs within the first 6 months of starting medication, and then the weight loss tends to level off. Most appetite suppressants are recommended only for short-term use – a few weeks to a few months – and not for more than one year continuously.

If you're considering appetite suppressant medication treatment, you should find out about potential risks. None of these medications come without their own set of potential side effects like irritability, sleeplessness, nervousness, dizziness and elevations in blood pressure and pulse. Sometimes it is recommended to take the last dose during the day to avoid trouble sleeping at night. All prescription diet medications are 'controlled substances', meaning doctors need to follow certain restrictions when prescribing them. Diet drugs are not 'magic bullets', or a one-shot fix. They won't take the place of normal dieting and exercise. Their major role is to help you start and stay on a diet and exercise plan, to lose weight and keep it off. Many studies have also shown that the majority of people who stop taking appetite suppressant medications regain the weight they had lost. Medications should be taken only under strict medical supervision, and not by buying online and self-treating.

fat blockers

The newest anti-obesity drugs have the ability to stop foods from turning into fat cells within the body. This class of drugs is called 'lipase inhibitors'.

They are different from other weight loss drugs in that they block the breakdown and absorption of fat from the gastrointestinal tract so it is not absorbed. Because they allow fat to be excreted in the stool, there are possible side effects, such as bloating, diarrhoea and flatulence. The

Diet medications

Drug	Brand name
Sibutramine	Meridia
Phentermine	Ionamin, Adepex P
Orlistat	Xenical
Benzphetamine	Didrex
Phendimetrazine	Plegine, Adipost, Bontril
Diethylpropion	Tenuate Dospan
Mazindol	Sanorex, Mazanor

Availability and drug brand names vary by country. Check with your doctor.

recommended dose is 3 times a day. Patients taking them are advised to take a supplement rich in the fat-soluble vitamins A, D, E and K, and to curtail their fat intake. While taking one of these drugs, if you eat high-fat foods, the side effects increase. If you eat a meal that contains no fat or skip a meal, a dose of medication may be skipped.

Natural pharmacy

We've all read the tempting claims; tablets that enable you to burn fat before food is digested, pills that help you to lose 2 dress sizes without dieting or exercise, and products that burn body fat while you sleep. Too bad that most of the marketing is simply not based on science. The list of 'natural' diet aids includes vitamins, minerals, herbs, botanicals, teas and other plant-derived substances, amino acids and concentrates, metabolites, constituents and extracts of these substances. For weight control, their general mode of action is to burn fat by increasing the basal metabolic rate, which translates to burning more calories. Other products work by enhancing your energy levels, assisting with digestion, reducing your appetite and easing water retention. Nutritional supplements are not required to undergo the rigorous testing that a drug is subjected to, so manufacturers are not asked to demonstrate that their product is either safe or effective. As a result, little is known about potential drug interactions, dosages and long-term effects. Some of these potent ingredients can overtax your heart, increase your blood pressure and cause other complications.

get thin quick

If it sounds too good to be true, it is, especially when it comes to diets in a capsule, pill or teacup. Supplements alone will never get you svelte. You have to do your part.

The key diet aid ingredients currently on the market:

Caffeine – a central nervous stimulant and a diuretic.

Chromium piccolinate – an essential mineral that is not made by the body and must be obtained from the diet. Important in the metabolism of fats and carbohydrates, chromium may increase fat loss and lean muscle gain.

Chitosan – derived from chitin, a polysaccharide found in the exoskeleton of shellfish such as shrimp, lobster and crabs. Chitosan has been shown to decrease fat absorption significantly. Once activated in the stomach, it supposedly binds to fatty acids. Because the body cannot digest Chitosan molecules, the fatty acids that are bound to it are eliminated from the large intestine without being absorbed by the body.

Citramax – highly concentrated extract of Gracinia Cambogia, a fruit indigenous to India with a high concentration of hydroxycitrate.

Creatine – serves as an energy reserve in muscle cells.

Ephedra – also called ephedrine alkaloids, Ma Huang and Chinese Ephedra; a naturally occurring caffeine-like ingredient used as an appetite suppressant.

BEAUTY BYTES:

To look up weight control supplements, log on to www.ephedra.com and www.webrx.com.

TOP TIP:

Check with your doctor before using any diet aids, especially if you are taking any prescription medication. Some ingredients may interact with serious side effects.

Guarana – contains guaranine, which is almost identical to caffeine and stimulates the central nervous system, increases metabolism and has a mild diuretic effect. It also has all the negative effects of caffeine including anxiety, insomnia and hyperactivity.

L-Carnitine – amino acid produced in the liver and kidneys and stored in the skeletal muscles and heart, as well as in sperm and in the brain; used to improve fat metabolism and muscular performance.

Phenylaline – amino acid used to help balance appetite.

Psyllium – a source of dietary fibre used to treat constipation and reduce cholesterol, which may help lessen the appetite and encourage weight loss.

Pyruvate – a modified form of the sugar molecule appears to enhance weight loss in adults who are eating a low-fat diet, by increasing the body's resting metabolic rate (the amount of energy used by the body when at rest).

Spirulina – blue-green algae that appears to help encourage weight loss; a good source of protein and essential fatty acids.

Many diet aids accelerate the heart rate, thus increasing blood pressure, and interfere with the heart's normal rhythm or cause stroke. Other side effects include nervousness, anxiety and insomnia. A study found that many fat reducing formulas showed large discrepancies between the content on the label and what was actually contained, which ranged from no active ingredients to dangerously high levels. If you have liver problems or take medications that can harm the liver, the US FDA advises that you ask a doctor before taking kava.

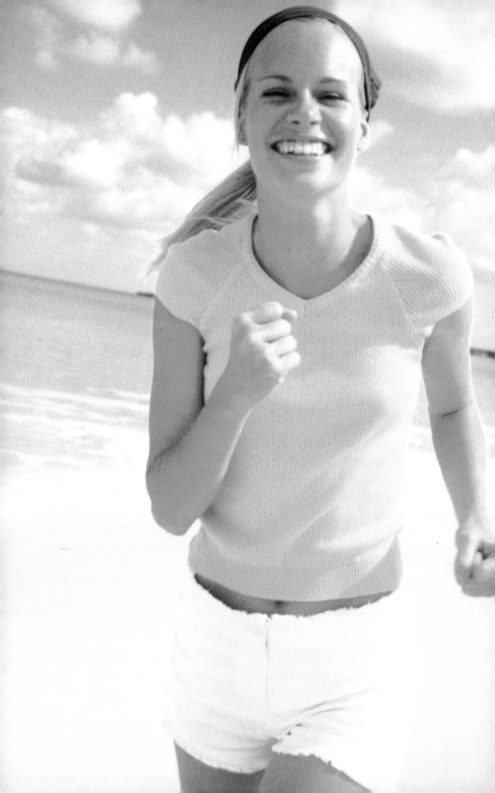

GET MOVING

GET MOVING

It shouldn't be a surprise that from your 20s, muscle mass and metabolism decline. Most women know that you can't eat the same way in your 40s as you did in your 20s and expect to stay trim. Activity levels also tend to decrease with age. If you have a slow metabolism to start out with, it becomes that much harder to maintain your size as you get older. Add a couple of pregnancies and hormonal changes to the mix, and you can see how much of an effort it takes to avoid piling on the pounds. As you age, you must be more careful about what you eat and watch your activity levels.

Even if you've never been to a gym, there is a workout suited to you, that can keep you trim as the years go by. If you've been inactive for too long, don't despair. Your muscles won't have gone to mush overnight. If you skip a week of exercise, you won't see much of a difference in your overall ability or strength. If you miss a month, you can expect to huff and puff a little more when you restart. If you skip 3 or 4 months, your body may need some retraining. Take it slowly - your aerobic strength and capability will have dropped a bit. If you've taken 6 months off, you'll be in the same cardiovascular shape as you were before you started exercising for the first time.

you go girl

If you're the type who makes empty promises about starting an exercise programme and sticking to it, there is still hope for you.

- **Have a check up** with your doctor if you're out of shape, *before* you begin any exercise programme.

- **Pace yourself** and learn how to breathe properly. Never exercise to the point of pain.

- **Hire a trainer** to force you to work out even when you're not in the mood, especially if you've paid for it already. Find an instructor who is certified and who you actually feel comfortable with and can afford. One solid hour with a professional is worth his/her weight in gold to get you on the right path.

BEAUTY BYTES:
Looking for a personal trainer? Log onto
www.ACEFitness.org, www.ACSN.org
or www.global-fitness.com.

Start a class that matches your ability level. Don't overtax yourself so that you can't keep up. If you're a beginner, there is no shame in saying so.

Get the right clothes; a pair of trainers, fabrics that can breathe, absorb sweat and feel comfortable without restricting your movement.

Find a partner and do it together. A companion can help keep you going when you're at the end of your rope.

Seek advice before you buy expensive exercise equipment. With today's assortment of tummy toners, heart rate monitors, treadmills, free weights and jogging strollers etc, it's hard to know what will work for you.

Get the timing right. If burning fat is your goal, doing cardio on an empty stomach after fasting all night may work best because you access your stored fat faster. Weight training first thing in the morning can increase your natural growth hormone levels. Some people are better off getting in a training session before work because they may be too tired at the end of the day. Others find that having a session or a run after a long day is ideal. The best time to do your routine, is when you have the time, energy and drive to enjoy it.

keeping it off

Exercise is the most effective treatment for fat reduction. Commiting to a regular exercise programme also gives you the best chance of losing weight and keeping it off.

Many women look at their overweight parents and come to the conclusion; I'm destined to be overweight and there's nothing I can do about it.' Some of us have genes that pre-dispose us to being overweight, and some overweight people may have an impaired metabolism that makes it harder, but neither of these facts preclude you from maintaining or losing weight.

Women who succeed incorporate behavioural strategies into their regime; learning about nutrition, planning what to eat and when and eating regular meals even between meetings and daily scheduling chaos. Exercise boosts weight loss because it builds muscle. Muscle tissue is the most metabolically active tissue in the body, so people with more muscles burn more calories, even when resting. It also increases your metabolic rate and keeps it elevated for a period even after you have finished your workout. Beyond boosting caloric

TOP TIP:
Don't weigh yourself everyday. Muscle is heavier than fat, so you won't see much change. Looking in the mirror and feeling your clothes getting looser are far more encouraging than the little number that registers on your bathroom scale. The best reward for losing a bit is treating yourself to a new outfit in a smaller size. Go for anything but food.

expenditure and moderating your appetite, exercise supports weight loss in other ways. It lowers your blood pressure, decreases your risk of diabetes and improves your cardiovascular system. It also serves to keep your self-esteem high, your spirits up and improves your overall body image. This sense of control contributes to reducing stress, which can trigger binge eating.

Exercise not only burns calories, but also improves glucose tolerance, which in turn moderates appetite. Glucose tolerance declines with excessive weight gain, making an extra carbohydrate load particularly destructive and increasing the likelihood of diabetes. Metabolic rate tends to decline after weight loss; when a large chunk of weight is lost quickly, more lean tissue is lost, which lowers your metabolic rate.

Use it to Lose it

Take advantage of every opportunity to be active; take the steps instead of the lift, walk instead of hailing a cab, walk briskly instead of strolling or park at the far end of the car park so you'll have to walk an extra 20 yards. Try to find some extra time in your day to sneak in a 15 minute jog or a quick aerobics class. Keep workout clothes in your office or car just in case the opportunity arises. At the end of the day, it all adds up.

Both weight training and cardiovascular exercise are essential. The more lean muscle tissue you have, the higher your resting metabolic rate will be. In other words, by developing more muscle, you will be burning more body fat all day long, even when you're not working out.

the bounce factor

Women have a smaller supply of the hormones that cause muscles to grow and develop, which is why men generally tend to be taller and more muscular.

Since we have more body fat, women typically have more fuel to burn off in endurance activities like running, cycling, swimming and hiking. Ideally, combine aerobic activity that increases the heart rate, with a resistance workout and weight training. Resistance exercise is good for muscle build-up, whereas aerobic exercise is better for reducing fat mass. Abdominal fat is most responsive to aerobics. Muscle fibres grow in response to the amount of work you make them do. If you're just starting to work with weights, anything you do will increase the amount of muscle you have on your frame. For example, you can do many repetitions at low resistance or fewer repetitions with more weight. As you get stronger, you can advance to the next level of resistance.

When it comes to burning off calories, people who do the same activity at the same pace for an equal amount of time can burn vastly different numbers of calories depending on their size. Generally, the larger you are, the more calories you burn, particularly from activities like walking or stair climbing where you have to carry your own weight. Fat oxidation works best if your activity level is continuous. Exercise should ideally be low impact, at about 50–70 per cent of cardiovascular endurance; for example, you should be breathless but still be able to talk while exercising.

lean on me

Resistance training builds up muscle and makes us stronger. Aerobic exercise stimulates the heart and increases the pulse rate. You need a little of both to get a proper workout.

When you start any new form of training, it will help your body improve. But if you carry on working out in exactly the same way using the same exercises, your body will adapt and stop improving at the same rate. Changing your workout routine will also keep it interesting. No matter what routine you follow, try to vary the intensity and duration of your workouts and the type of activities you do to get consistently good results. Using the proper technique will also ensure the best results from your programme. Not doing your exercises in the right way won't help. Learn a few different ways to exercise each muscle group in case you can't get to the machine you want to use at the gym. To keep your workout effective and efficient, choose exercises that simultaneously work several major muscle groups. Your equipment should be easily accessible. Working out becomes a chore if you have to drive far to the gym.

REALITY CHECK:
Pick a starting point and aim for 30 minutes a day, 5 days a week – the minimum recommended by medical experts. You can begin with 3 days a week at low intensities and work your way up gradually. Ideally, exercise should be done 7 days a week. Doing something as simple as walking for 30 minutes every day will help control your body weight.

tipping the scales

Exercise improves glucose tolerance, which in turn moderates appetite. Glucose tolerance declines with excessive weight gain, making an extra carb load particularly destructive.

Metabolism is the body's process of converting substances ingested into the body to other compounds. Sugar makes insulin levels go mad, causing metabolism to shut down. This makes the body store more fat. Losing a lot of weight quickly means a large amount of lean tissue is lost, thus lowering the rate of metabolism. Losing weight without exercising could mean you are sacrificing muscle mass. Severely restrictive diets can reduce the metabolic rate by up to 30 per cent. Strengthening exercises are critical to losing and maintaining weight. They help preserve muscle and bone, boosting your metabolism. Because muscle burns calories and fat doesn't, having a high level of lean muscle mass in your body and a low amount of fat means you will burn more calories, both during physical activity and when sitting in a chair, cooking dinner or sleeping.

The energy used to keep the body alive (basal metabolism) accounts for 50–75 per cent of daily caloric expenditure. Day-to-day activities burn 15–40 per cent of calories. All physical activity burns calories, even walking to the fridge. The number of calories you burn generally depends on your body composition, metabolism and food intake.

BEAUTY BYTES:

To get help starting an exercise programme, visit www.nutricise.com or www.4woman.org.

Certain activities burn calories more quickly than others. This is relative to the exercise. For example, you might go running for an hour, whereas you would perhaps only do push-ups for a few minutes at a time. The figures given below refer to somebody weighing 67 kg.

Aerobic

Fast dancing
9 calories per minute

Kickboxing
7.5 calories per minute

Step aerobics
12 calories per minute

Aerobic class
6.5 calories per minute

Skipping
7 calories per minute

Jogging (5.5 mph)
8 calories per minute

Running (10 mph)
17.6 calories per minute

Cycling
6.6 calories per minute

Resistance

Sports climbing
6 calories per minute

Push-ups (vigorous effort)
9.4 calories per minute

Push-ups (moderate effort)
5.3 calories per minute

Sit-ups
5.3 calories per minute

Weight lifting (vigorous effort)
7 calories per minute

Weight lifting (moderate effort)
3.5 calories per minute

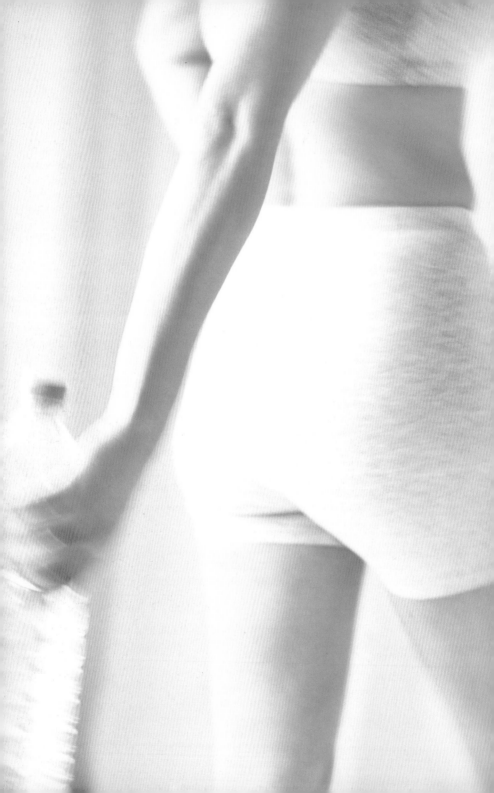

THE WAR ON DIMPLES

THE WAR ON DIMPLES

What does every woman over 20 have behind her? Cellulite. Although it's normal, the bad news is that there is no cure. An estimated 80-90 per cent of women have some form of cellulite. The many causes begin with the usual suspects like genetics, hormones, nutrition, stress and smoking and include excess fat, crash dieting and rapid weight gain. Even sleeping pills, diuretics and diet pills have been cited.

Cellulite lives in the subcutaneous layer of the skin. It varies in thickness and is laced with fat cells held in place by a network of fibres that cushions the muscles and organs. When all is well, waste products are removed and smooth curves result. When fats, fluids and toxins are trapped deep in the skin, the tissue thickens and hardens, giving a dimpling effect. As we mature, the outer layer of the skin thins so the dimples become more obvious. The most cellulite-prone areas are the buttocks and thighs. Cellulite is most visible when you are standing. Topical agents, packs, wraps, massage and ultrasound may offer temporary improvement, but there is no scientifically proven treatment that gets rid of it permanently. Reducing cellulite takes commitment.

the bottom line

Cellulite is not necessarily a factor of body weight. All women know that you don't have to be heavy to have cellulite.

Although diet and lifestyle do affect cellulite formation, a large part of the problem is caused by the build-up of toxins and fat. Cellulite can affect any woman, regardless of size, weight and body type. At some point, whether you're a size 8 or 16, if you're female, you're likely to see a skin pattern developing that looks a little like quilting, and I don't mean the kind on Chanel bags. It starts on the back of your thighs, extends to the buttocks and eventually travels to the dreaded saddlebags, the fronts of the thighs, buttocks, knees and upper abdomen. This is cellulite and it has been known to reduce grown women to tears.

Oestrogen production makes cellulite unique to women. Any fluctuation in hormone levels contributes to fat storage in the fat cells. As they expand to make room for extra fat, connective fibres are pulled down and fat cells bulge out. The skin is connected to the underlying structures by vertical fibrous bands, which act like buttons on a mattress, blocking the drainage of lymph fluid. As the trapped lymph fluid collects, the fibres get tighter and these areas of skin balloon up, causing dimpling of the skin. All of these factors together create the dreaded 'orange peel' effect. Exercise is vital for achieving proper circulation, which combats cellulite formation and keeps your body toned. It also works to relieve tension and keep you stress-free. Tension stresses the muscles and causes the connective tissue that covers the muscles to seize up and block the tissues, preventing efficient waste elimination. Correct breathing and relaxation can ease your tension, oxygenate the body and help with the body's natural purification process. The better your body functions, the more effectively it can eliminate the toxins that can cause cellulite.

eating patterns

A good way to start fighting cellulite is by detoxing, which means adding foods that are easiest for the body to break down, use and get rid of, and subtracting anything that inhibits that process.

Drink 2–3 litres of water a day to assist your body in getting rid of unwanted toxins and waste. The message is; be good to your liver and it will metabolize fats more efficiently so you'll be less likely to develop the dreaded 'C' word.

- **DOs** Fresh fruits • Vegetables • Whole grain foods • Low fat • High fibre • Complex carbohydrates • Water

- **DON'Ts** Chocolate • Caffeine • Fizzy drinks • Alcohol • Sugar • Starches • Salt • Spices • Animal fats • Dairy • White flour • Processed foods • Fried foods

If your goal is to audition for 'Baywatch', you need to hire a nutritionist, personal chef and trainer to design a diet and fitness programme and keep you on it. It wouldn't hurt to stay out of bistros, pubs and cafes either. Beware of diet saboteurs; people who may mean well but encourage you to treat yourself to dessert or bring you chocolates as a reward for losing a few pounds.

TOP TIP:
Avoid the 'ine's' –
caffeine, nicotine, wine,
saccharine, margarine,
theobromine
(chocolate)

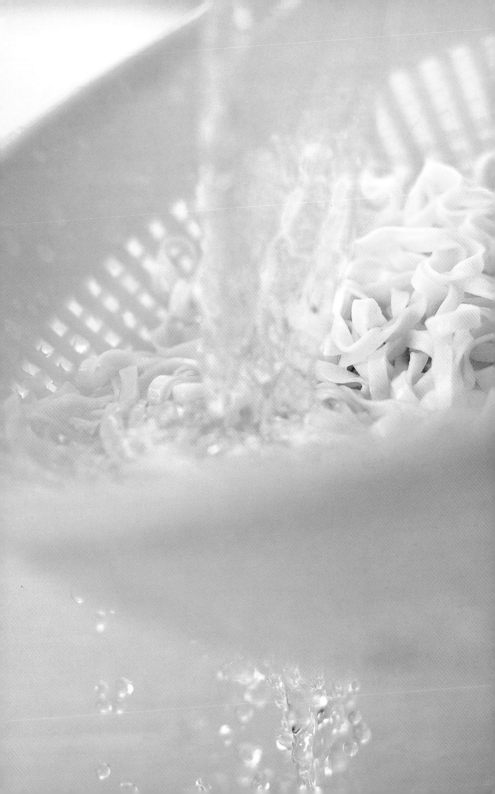

heavenly bodies

Cellulite may seem more ominous than regular fat but it is just arranged differently. Weight loss and exercise will minimize cellulite but you can still have lumps and bumps.

Kneading me

Massage techniques increase the circulation of blood and flow of lymph, a milky white fluid that carries impurities and waste out of the tissues. The oxygen capacity of the blood can increase by as much as 10–15 per cent after vigorous massage. By manipulating the muscles, therapeutic massage stimulates the circulatory and lymphatic systems that break down fatty tissue. The lymph fluid does not circulate throughout the body as blood does, so it has to be moved around by putting pressure on the muscles so they contract. When you are still, the muscles contract less and consequently fail to stimulate lymph flow on their own. The Swiss method of manual lymphatic drainage is widely used to speed up toxin elimination. This has an instant but temporary, slimming effect. This technique can be used all over the body, from the face and neck down to the ankles, where fluid tends to settle. Deep tissue massage can also be useful in reducing cellulite by targeting areas that are difficult to stimulate with exercise, such as the inner knee and upper thigh. Try simply massaging each leg in circular movements for a couple of minutes each day to break down fat and get rid of toxins.

BEAUTY BYTE:
For more about massage techniques visit
www.amtamassage.org

Skin-fold rolling

Endermologie®, the skin-fold rolling technology developed in France and introduced to the US in 1991, can temporarily reduce the appearance of cellulite. The operative word is temporarily. Endermologie® is not the total answer; it is one part of a multi-pronged approach to slimming and toning. A rolling, suction movement is applied with a hand held computer head that smoothes the skin surface, and stimulates circulation by eliminating toxins in the tissues. Most women report that they feel energized and relaxed after each session. Before you begin the treatment, you will slip into a sheer, white nylon leotard that runs from your neck to your ankles. For some strange reason, it only comes in white, possibly to make your fat cells stand out. Trust me, once you see yourself in this body stocking, you are sure to sign on for lifetime membership. The treatment usually begins with the therapist working on the back, then the calves, buttocks, thighs, feet, backs of the arms and on to the neck and face with a smaller handpiece. The focus is on cellulite-prone areas like the tummy, saddlebags and front and backs of the thighs. Even on a relatively low setting, you can feel the power of suction. Few women ever get up to the highest levels unless they are into self-punishment. After a series of 40-minute sessions once or twice per week for 16–20 weeks, be prepared for monthly maintenance or you can kiss your progress goodbye. Endermologie® doesn't take away excess fat or any dress sizes. It works well as an adjunct to body liposuction, to smooth and tone the skin once the fat cells are removed. It has been shown to speed up the healing process. Combining Endermologie® with ultrasound or sound waves may deliver better results that last longer on some thighs. There are no guarantees.

Thalassotherapy

Original thalassotherapy involves the use of sea water and sea air pumped from the ocean. Many products and treatments in spas today are designed to recreate the benefits of the thalassotherapy experience. Ocean-derived ingredients include seaweed, sea minerals and sea mud. Seaweed and algae saturated with mineral salts, trace elements and amino acids are known for their rejuvenative properties and have long been used for weight loss and many ailments. With the properties of human plasma, seaweed absorbs nutrients of the sea, which transfer to the body when placed on the skin. Seaweeds are excellent sources of several vitamins, pantothenic acid, folic acid, niacin and iodine. Research suggests that they are rich in minerals, especially potassium, calcium, magnesium, phosphorus, iron, zinc and manganese. The treatments help encourage the body to eliminate waste materials, reduce excess water retention and improve circulation.

Shrink wrap

Body wraps are commonly found on the menu of spa treatments for invigorating and detoxifying the skin. The body is usually swathed for up to an hour in mineral-rich mud, herbs and/or seaweed-soaked cloths that aid in circulation and work to firm body contours. You can expect to be wrapped from your chest to your toes and even your arms while lying on a thermal blanket to keep you warm and cozy. A technician then unwraps you and for the finishing touch, a body massage may be done to enhance circulation and encourage oxygen to flow to blocked tissues.

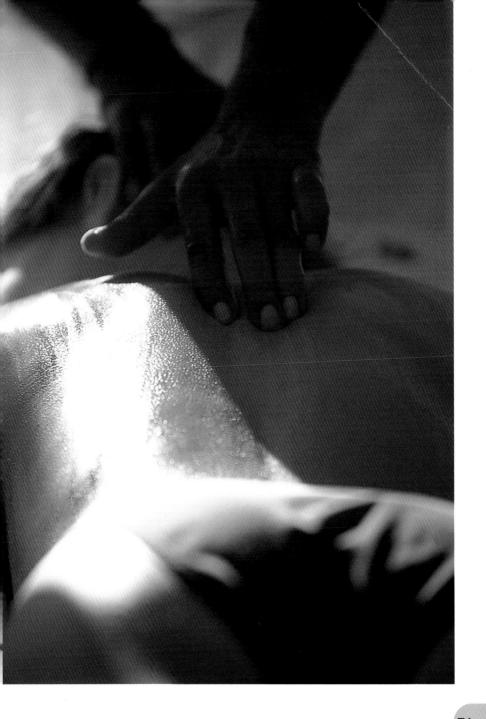

Dry brushing

Dry skin brushing is a method used to remove dried, dead cells that block the pores of the skin. This allows the skin to breathe more easily and increases its ability to protect and eliminate the waste produced by metabolism. Dry brushing can also improve the texture and appearance of the skin. It should be done using a natural bristle body brush, a horsehair or nylon bristle brush or a glove, before taking a bath or shower. Skin brushing for a couple of minutes will boost circulation. Start with the lower limbs, arms and back, then the front of the body, brushing the skin in an upward movement towards the heart using a moderate pressure and short strokes. If you have a soft brush, the face can be done as well, using circular motions. The benefits of dry brushing are that it stimulates and increases blood circulation in all organs and tissues, especially capillaries near the skin. It aids the skin in ridding the system of toxins, placing less of a burden on the organs and nerve endings in the skin, and rejuvenates the entire nervous system. It can reduce cellulite deposits, tones and tightens the skin, increases resistance to colds and improves overall health. It improves clarity of thought by stimulating the lungs and increasing the oxygen supply to the brain and actually improves thinking. Doing this daily before your shower helps revitalize the body and improve the skin's appearance.

Mesotherapy

The technique of Mesotherapy was developed by Dr Pistor in 1958 in France, to stimulate the mesoderm, or middle layer of the skin, using injections. The fibrous connective tissues, cartilage, bone, muscle and fat make up the mesoderm layer. Natural plant extracts are used with a combination of agents like enzymes and nutrients to stimulate venous and lymph flow. Some doctors use a solution containing a vasodilator, which increases blood flow and stimulates lymph drainage, and a lipolytic agent to break down fat tissue. An anaesthetic may also be used. Mesotherapy injections are given to improve the venous and lymphatic flow and also to break down the fat nodules. Extremely small needles are used, which just penetrate the body superficially, typically 4–6 millimetres. The treatments are usually given once per week. As improvement is seen, the procedure may be repeated less frequently, such as once every 2 weeks or once a month. For long-term chronic conditions such as cellulite, at least 15 sessions of Mesotherapy will be needed and the process should be repeated as the cellulite returns.

Mesotherapy is undertaken to avoid oral medications that have to go through the bloodstream to get to the area of the body that needs treatment. Droplets of the same medication are introduced through multiple micro-injections at or around the point of trouble, never deeper than subcutaneous or intradermally. It must be performed by a licenced health care clinician who is permitted to do injections.

Creams, pills and snake oil

Anti-cellulite creams have been touted to help reduce and prevent the appearance of cellulite by improving the elasticity of the skin. They claim to do everything from strengthening to renewing and softening. In conjunction with increased circulation and a change of diet and lifestyle, some of these products do work, by strengthening the network of connective tissue. Supplements containing caffeine, ginkgo biloba, evening primrose oil and fish oils among other ingredients, have never been scientifically proven to have any systemic effect on cellulite. Dietary supplements are not regulated as long as they pose no unreasonable risk and are not sold as a cure for a disease or medical condition, so marketing campaigns for cellulite cures are virtually unrestricted.

Topical creams and gels can be safely used to temporarily reduce the appearance of cellulite. Many of these contain intense moisturizers that make skin feel softer and more supple, and alpha hydroxy acids (AHAs) to exfoliate dead skin cells and create a smoother, less bumpy appearance. Botanical ingredients like ivy extract, capsicum, black pepper extract, cinnamon, ginger, green tea and mandarin, are sometimes used to improve microcirculation. Aminophylline and caffeine have been used to stimulate vascular flow into the fat. Wild yam, omega-3, lineolic acid and evening primrose oil have been used to stimulate hormones in the skin. Topical retinols have also been shown to have an effect on cellulite by stimulating blood flow to the dermal fat. The downside is that once you stop using any of these creams, the skin returns to its original state since they cannot permanently alter the skin's natural properties.

dos and don'ts

The secret to smooth curves is a combination of diet, exercise and therapies. Cellulite treatments should accompany a comprehensive programme aimed at improving metabolism.

- **DO** expect cellulite to become more noticeable with age as the connective tissue becomes stiffer and the skin holding the fat in place gets looser.

- **DO** drink 6–8 glasses of water daily. Poor lymphatic flow, due to lack of physical activity and inadequate water intake, is a big contributor.

- **DO** avoid alcohol. Even though cellulite may drive you to drink, it can pile on pounds and keep you bloated.

- **DON'T** forget to exfoliate daily with AHAs or lactic acid creams, and use a loofah or massage brush in the shower for stimulation.

- **DON'T** waste money on electro-stimulation treatments – join a gym, buy a dog to run in the park with, or hire a trainer.

- **DON'T** have liposuction solely as a means to get rid of cellulite. Your body will look better, but it won't be dimple-free.

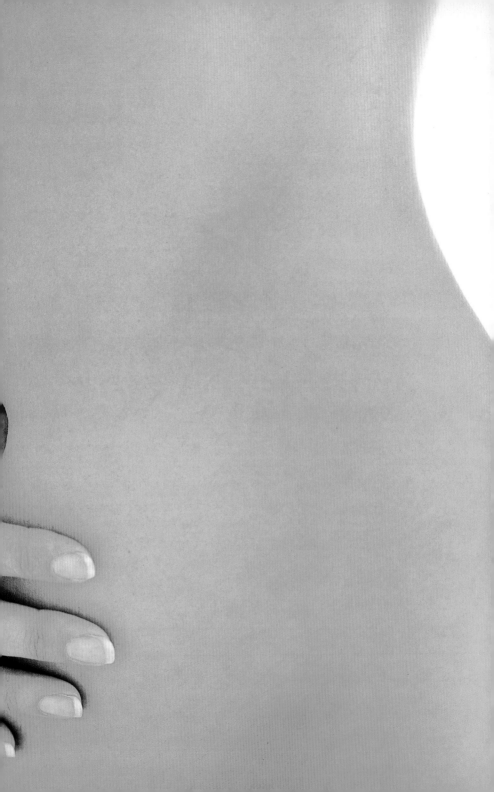

BODY CONTOURING

You go to the gym 3 times a week and watch what you eat, but you still feel like the rear end of a bus. Liposuction is a safe, effective way to remove unsightly bulges, giving you an improved shape and contour. This explains why liposuction or 'lipoplasty' has long been the most popular cosmetic surgical procedure, worldwide. In 2001, according to the American Society for Aesthetic Plastic Surgery, 385,000 lipoplasty procedures were performed in the US alone. For women striving for a better body, getting rid of unwanted fat cells sounds like a dream come true. Picture this; you go to sleep with fatty bulges and when you awake, they're gone!

Adult fat cells are thought to be incapable of multiplying. As you gain weight they expand and as you lose weight they contract, but the number and distribution stay the same. This accounts for why thin women still complain about localized fatty deposits that won't budge. Liposuction reduces your overall number of fat cells and changes your shape, so any future weight gain or loss won't be as noticeable in the areas that were treated. It can jumpstart a serious weight loss and exercise programme, or you can think of it as a treat after you've done your part to reshape your body.

a girl's best friend

You can still gain weight after liposuction, but if you do, it will mostly be in areas not suctioned, since the normal number of fat cells are still there and will continue to expand.

Be aware that there are still fat cells in the areas that were suctioned, so those body parts are not off limits. The good news is that if you do gain fat in areas of the body that weren't your primary trouble spots, it is usually very responsive to diet and exercise. For example, if you have liposuction on your worst area and you gain half a stone afterwards, it may show up on your hips instead. When you lose that half a stone, it will go quicker from the hips because it was the last place the fat was gained.

Liposuction is not a miracle cure and it can't give you the body of a supermodel. Before having liposuction, your cosmetic surgeon should discuss your lifestyle, aerobic shape and body weight fluctuations. If you have a history of an eating disorder like bulimia, anorexia, binge eating, or have been on prescription weight control medications, tell your surgeon in advance.

These procedures are for anyone who cannot obtain the trim and properly contoured look that they are after with diet and exercise, and possess good skin elasticity. They would not be suitable for someone who is looking to lose large volumes of weight. Patients who exceed their ideal body weight by over 30 per cent may only be candidates for limited fat removal because of safety concerns and should undergo these

YES IT CAN

- Remove fat deposits
- Change your shape
- Take out fat from beneath the skin

NO IT CAN'T

- Cure cellulite
- Tighten loose skin
- Take out fat from underneath muscles

procedures in stages. Those who weigh over 50 per cent more than their dream weight should seek other remedies for weight loss as an initial step.

Some areas of the body have fatty deposits that tend to stick around no matter how much you starve yourself or how many metres you run, sit-ups you do, or laps you swim. Fat deposits that don't respond to the usual exercise and diet regimes are ideal targets for liposuction. If you are only overweight in certain areas of your body, for example, you have saddlebags, you would have to lose a large amount of weight in order to shrink the size of your thighs. The weight will come off from everywhere including the breasts and face, and not just directly where you need it most. The beauty of liposuction surgery is that it will just focus on your chosen areas.

Typically, women in their 20s and 30s, go for liposuction of their inner and outer thighs and knees. In the 40s and 50s, in addition to the thighs, the abdomen, hips, waist and upper back become popular due to gaining weight with each child. Extra weight gained in your peri-menopausal years tends to settle around your mid section. By age 60, the hips and bottom spread and liposuction procedures give way to body lifts as skin thins and elasticity is lost.

outer limits

Every woman alive who has ever had liposuction has complained to her cosmetic surgeon; 'Doctor, couldn't you have taken a little more fat out?'

The ideal liposuction patient will be at or close to a normal weight. The best 'pre-lipo' weight is one you can maintain without starving yourself. Most doctors will not perform liposuction on patients who are 2 stone or more overweight, or over 30 per cent more than their ideal body weight. If you're just 1 stone away from a size that is acceptable to you, lose some weight before surgery and more after. If you put on a few pounds after lipo, you'll blow your investment. If you lose some, your result will look that much better. It is not uncommon to have a small touch-up procedure 6 months later.

There are limits as to how many areas can be operated on and how much fat can be removed, based on your size, weight and tolerance to surgery. With new techniques, amounts of 5–10 pounds of fat and fluids can be removed at one stage, depending on your size at the start. If there are several areas you want suctioned, you can easily reach that level rather quickly. If there is too much for one stage, the surgeon may suggest that you lose weight before having liposuction. When skin elasticity is not ideal, a staged procedure is a good solution. The liposuction would be done first, and if you don't get enough skin contraction, then skin excision and internal tightening can be done at a later date, as in a tummy tuck or a thigh lift. In certain selected cases, up to 10–20 pounds of fat may be suctioned, which is categorized as large volume lipoplasty, and is considered far more risky.

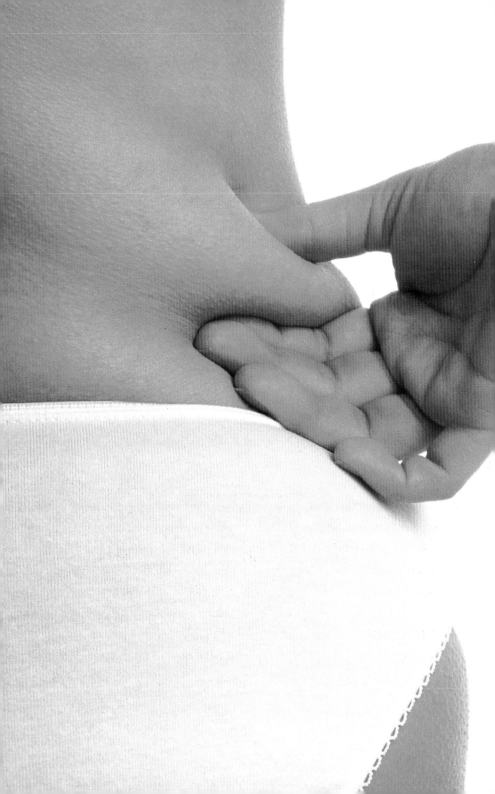

the art of liposuction

Liposuction has come a long way since its introduction in the mid 1970s. Modern techniques are vastly improved for women who want to make their fat cells history.

The procedure is very straightforward. The surgeon uses cannulae – hollow, tubular instruments with holes at one end to trap the fat. The cannula is attached to suction tubing through which the excess fat is evacuated. These instruments come in various shapes, lengths and sizes depending on the thickness and location of the fat. They have highly polished surfaces to slip through the fatty tissues with minimum friction or damage, so there is less bruising. The instruments are typically blunt-tipped to prevent cutting through the skin, and fat is suctioned out through strategically placed holes at the tip. Traditional liposuction relies on the mechanical disruption of fat cells by the movement of the cannula and the vacuum of the suction pump. Tiny incisions are made at the sites where fat is to be removed, and a wetting solution is infused to provide a numbing effect, reduce bleeding and improve fat extraction. Cannulae are inserted under the skin, moved in a back and forth and criss-cross fashion within the fat and then the fat is vacuumed away. The size of the cannulae used can affect the smoothness of the skin after liposuction. The use of large cannulae tends to create irregularities more often than cannulae of less than 3 mm in diameter.

The output of fat is measured and the patient is checked for symmetry, although most of us have one side that is naturally slightly fuller than the other. The procedure is completed when a safe level of fat removal is achieved. You are then monitored closely to make sure you have received enough fluid hydration and are able to tinkle without difficulty. After tumescent liposuction, some blood-tinged local anaesthetic solution remains under the skin. This excess fluid is either slowly absorbed into the blood stream or rapidly removed by draining through skin incisions. Rapid drainage reduces postoperative pain, swelling and bruising. Surgery can be performed in hospital or at an accredited office surgery centre. For larger procedures, staying in the hospital or clinic overnight may be recommended.

New studies have shown that liposuction may provide additional health benefits for some women. A dramatic reduction in body weight can be useful as a stepping stone to a long term weight loss programme. Large volume liposuction (the removal of more than 10 lbs or 5 quarts of fat) may also lead to a lowering of blood pressure and insulin levels in some women who are more than 50 lbs above their ideal weight. Strict postop monitoring is vital after aggressive liposuction procedures.

TOP TIP:
The larger the volume of fat and fluids removed from the body, the more risky the procedure becomes and the longer the recovery is likely to be.

fat traps

Technological advances in liposuction techniques have greatly improved the results you can expect and made it safer, faster and more effective than ever.

Tumescent

Tumescent anaesthesia has had a significant impact on liposuction. Since 1987, it has virtually eliminated the need for blood transfusions, as very little blood is lost during surgery. A warmed, diluted sterile solution containing lidocaine, epinephrine and intravenous fluid is injected into the area to be treated. As the liquid enters the fat, it becomes swollen, firm and blanched. There is the 'wet', and the 'superwet' technique, referring to the amount of fluid injected. The expanded fat compartments allow the liposuction cannula to travel smoothly beneath the skin as the fat is removed. Saline softens the fat, adrenaline decreases the bruising and the anaesthetic provides pain relief. For small amounts of fat, tumescent solution may be the only anaesthetic given. The anaesthetic in the solution can also be supplemented with sedatives to make you relaxed and sleepy during the procedure. General anaesthetic may be used for larger procedures involving multiple areas.

Ultrasound

Internal: Ultrasonic energy was first used in liposuction in 1995. This is a 2 stage procedure. First, ultrasonic sound waves, like shock waves, are transmitted into the fatty tissues from the tip of a fine probe. Ultrasonic energy is used to liquefy or melt the fat, which is then removed using a cannula and a low-pressure vacuum. Ultrasonic liposuction is often used for large volumes and multiple areas and is good for areas where the deep fat is thicker and harder to get out; e.g. back rolls and upper abdomen. It is usually combined with traditional liposuction when both the deeper and the more superficial fat is being removed. When previous liposuction has been done, it may be useful to soften the resulting scar tissue, to make it easier for the surgeon to remove the fat. Some patients report a slight burning sensation after surgery.

External: External ultrasonic energy, used for years by physical therapists, was introduced in 1997 for use in lower frequencies to soften fat deposits and smooth out bumps on the skin's surface. It is also used after liposuction to break up the hard spots and lumpiness, especially around the tummy.

Vaser: This new ultrasound technology utilizes bursts of ultrasonic energy to break up fat cells for removal. Smaller, more delicate probes are used to increase the surgeon's precision and the safety of the procedure.

Power trip

In 1998, the use of power was introduced to fat sucking methods. The cannulae used are motor-driven so they vibrate as they work, which makes removing fat easier and faster for the surgeon. The reciprocating frequency provides enough energy through the tip of the instruments to glide through fatty tissue. Since less physical exertion is required, many surgeons report that they can get better results and remove more fat. Postoperative pain, bruising and swelling may also be reduced with this method.

risky business

The risks from liposuction are actually very small. When they do occur, they are most often related to the expertise of the surgeon or the anaesthetist.

Specific risks from the tumescent technique (see page 64) include rare complications like pulmonary oedema – a collection of fluid in the lungs – which may occur if too much fluid is administered, and lidocaine toxicity, which can occur if there is too much lidocaine in the solution. If the surgeon injects too much of the solution, there is a risk that you could be drowning in fluids. Overworking the heart is a possible consequence. There is also the possibility of causing a fat embolism, which is when a piece of fat travels into the bloodstream. This can cause serious problems. Anti-embolism boots are often used during surgery to prevent a blood clot from forming in the deep veins of the pelvis or legs. The risk of a seroma – an oozing or pooling of clear serum – is possible in certain areas like the abdomen, after ultrasound techniques have been used. In these cases, the surgeon may drain the excess fluid to relieve pressure. The other risks apply to any surgical procedure and include infection, bleeding, skin loss and nerve damage. All of these are rare. Generally, the greater the volume of fat and fluids removed, the higher the chances of having a problem.

Choosing a cosmetic surgeon

Questions to ask

What can I reasonably expect as a final result?

Where will the surgery be performed?

How long will the procedure take?

How much do you expect my skin to contract after the fat is removed?

What kind of anaesthesia is used, and what credentials does the person administering it have?

How will you manage fluid balance during the procedure?

How will my recovery be monitored immediately after surgery?

How long have you been performing this procedure, and how many times have you performed it in the last twelve months?

What percentage of patients have had significant complications?

If the procedure has to be repeated or corrected, should I expect to be charged again? (The surgeon should provide you with his/her policy on revisions for liposuction and bodylifts.)

What should I expect postoperatively, in terms of soreness, medication, bathing and level of activity?

Ask to see photos of recent patients whose body type is similar to yours, before and after they had their surgery.

liposculpture

Liposculpture is a superficial variation on liposuction whereby smaller amounts of fat are removed and reinjected to create improved contour.

Liposculpture, also called syringe liposculpture, was introduced in the mid 1980s. It uses fine instruments to remove small amounts of fat to define features, accentuate muscles and sharpen the appearance of the neck, cheeks, abdomen, buttocks, calves and ankles. Superficial liposuction techniques remove tiny bits of fat just under the surface of the skin, and fat injections may be used to fill in contour defects. Some cosmetic surgeons gently break down adhesions and cellulite deposits by cutting through the fibrous tissues using V-shaped instruments.

Combined with a layer of injected fat, this technique smooths out irregularities. Since liposuction became popular, surgeons have used progressively smaller instruments, so it is now a more delicate procedure. The really good surgeons can reshape your contours in a very subtle way, causing minimal trauma to the tissues.

TOP TIP:

Look at your body naked in a full-length mirror. Evaluate each part separately – the upper abdomen, lower abdomen, legs, etc. To achieve the most attractive curves possible, focus on the areas you would benefit most from having recontoured. For example, if your thighs bulge, liposuctioning just one part like the outer portion, may make the inner thighs or hips look too large in comparison.

body parts

Almost any body part can be suctioned for better contour and reduced volume, from the face all the way down to the ankles.

The most popular areas for women are the abdomen, inner and outer thighs, hips, flanks and knees. The trend is to treat areas of the body circumferentially, instead of removing fat deposits from selected spots. Sections like the abdomen, hips, waist, and all around the thighs and knees, and upper arms, are combined to maximize the potential for skin to shrink afterwards. It is not rare to have liposuction done in stages; for example, the lower body in one go and the trunk later. Liposuction can even be used to reduce large breasts in women whose breasts have a lot of fatty tissue.

Ab flab

Generally speaking, the springier your skin is, the better liposuction works. If your greatest concern is flabby skin due to pregnancy, ageing or yo-yo dieting, liposuction can actually make it look worse. Some fatty areas are less forgiving to major fat removal than others and more often lead to sagging skin; for example, upper arms, inner thighs, knees, abdomen and the neck, in women. If your ultimate goal is to be taut and super trim from the waist down, a tummy tuck, thigh lift, or lower body lift are the only viable options. These involve tightening underlying muscles and removing and redraping excess skin. Unfortunately, they leave significant scarring and the recovery period is longer, but the results can be amazing.

The right to bare arms

Some call them 'batwings'; those dreaded flabby arms can really hurt someone if they swing when you wave goodbye. Along with inner thighs, upper arms are the pet hate of more women than we can count. If you're longing to go sleeveless, read on. Intensive upper extremity exercises with weight training help greatly, but after a certain age or if gravity has taken a toll on the thin skin of the arms, improvement won't be dramatic or quick. If you have good, elastic skin, liposuction can be the answer to your prayers. Plastic surgeons can recontour the upper arm by taking out fat through tiny incisions around the elbow. You won't end up with perfectly toned, defined arms, but you may be able to go sleeveless with pride. The skin contracts to a better shape after about 3 weeks, when the bruising and most of the swelling has gone. After about 3 months, you can see the final contour change.

Rubber tyres

Particularly in women who have had children and those in the perimenopausal range (from the age of 35 onwards), fat deposits tend to accumulate in the middle section of the body. If you can't remember the last time you had a waist and your hips seem to have a mind of their own, liposuction may be able to help bring you back into belt-donning shape. The upper and lower tummy, waist, hips and flanks can be suctioned to reduce girth. It is not a substitute for a full tummy tuck or abdominoplasty, but most women in reasonably good health and firmness, can get some skin shrinkage. If it is a washboard flat stomach you crave, then a more invasive surgery, which tightens the muscles and removes excess skin, is in order.

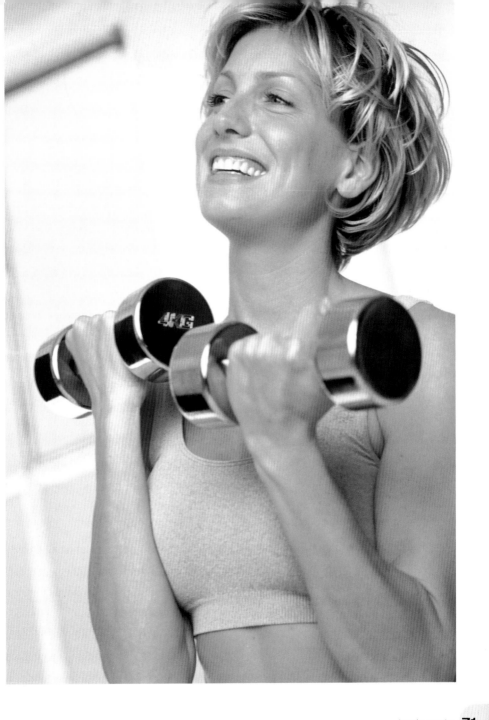

Thigh zone

What one woman calls her buttocks, a cosmetic surgeon might refer to as her 'lateral thighs' or 'banana rolls' – the fold of skin and fat just below the buttock crease. Another issue for women is that of how each part of the anatomy flows into the next, for example, how the buttocks are connected to the hips and outer thighs. The topic of rear ends is about contour and proportions; i.e. the transition from the trunk to the buttocks should be smooth and the latter should appear as though they belong to the rest of your body, instead of having a life of their own. Improving the backside involves taking out and putting in, fat that is. Liposuction can be done for hips, thighs and banana rolls, but is rarely recommended near the buttock crease because removing the fat can actually increase sagging. The best candidates are women who are a size 10 on top and a 14 on bottom. If you have a small backside with protruding thighs, recontouring only the buttocks may make the thighs look that much bigger. They are usually done as a set. Fat from other body parts can be sucked out and injected back to smooth out your gluteus maximus, fill out dents and add curves. If you're waifish everywhere else, you may be stuck with a flat rear.

TOP TIP:

If you have had scoliosis or any type of hip injury, one side may appear higher than the other.

A leg up

Getting your legs fit to bare can be high maintenance. Flabby knees are the bane of any woman's existence, and all the crunches and squats on earth won't make them go away significantly if that is your problem spot. Many women think they have Miss Piggy knees, when in fact; it is their joints that make their knees look large and not fat at all. Liposuction can be used to delicately recontour legs from the ankles, calves and knees up to the inner and outer thighs, taking inches off the circumference of the leg. Fatty deposits can in many cases be suctioned away from the inner portion of the knees. The flabby pouches on the front of the knees are not really ideal for reduction by liposuction. Calves are tricky because they are often largely muscle, but suctioning even small amounts can make a big difference to the overall shape. Liposuction of the legs takes longer than other areas to fully settle down, because swelling tends to travel downward and rest below the knee. This is one procedure that is usually best left for colder months when you can easily cover up bruising and swelling by wearing trousers, long skirts and opaque tights. Scars are hidden and tiny, so they won't give your secret away.

recovery

Speedy healing has made the popularity of liposuction soar. You can be back at work after a long weekend. In a couple of weeks, you'll be ready for bathing suit season.

Generally, patients experience significant swelling for 2 days following the procedure, but this rapidly subsides, and resolves quickly over the next few weeks. You should look good after 3 weeks and continue to improve over the next 3–6 months. Bruising is usually minimal and showering is permitted after 2 days. Many women return to work or some activity within 2–4 days for small liposuctions, 10–14 days for more extensive procedures. Many resume an exercise programme in 2 weeks. Postop pain is minimal, especially with an expertly administered anaesthetic. You will see your new shape best after 3 weeks, when most of the swelling has subsided. After 6 months, the final contour will be visible. If you are having thighs, knees or ankles done, keeping your legs elevated will reduce the swelling faster.

A major benefit of liposuction is that the scars left are tiny, less than half an inch. Small slit-like scars can be placed in hidden areas like the belly button, the crease under the buttocks and inside the knee. These generally heal brilliantly and they are rarely a problem, even in the teeniest, tiniest thong. After surgery, a compression garment will be applied that looks like a cross between a corset out of the set of Moulin Rouge and granny's undergarments. Wearing the girdle for a few weeks will hold everything in and keep swelling to a minimum. Most women actually feel better with some compression and wear the girdle or support hose for longer.

honey I shrunk

After liposuction, most women find that they have a better shape with fewer bulges. Clothes that were snug around the hips and thighs will flow nicely without pulling and stretching.

- You will weigh more right after liposuction than before surgery. Your face, feet and hands will swell up from all the fluids pumped into you.

- Swelling travels down like everything else, so don't be surprised if you're puffy and bruised in places you didn't have suctioned.

- Warm aromatic baths infused with lavender and rosemary can soothe and relax sore body parts.

- Use a lubricant like petrolatum, polysporin or Vitamin E oil to keep incisions soft and stop scabs from forming. Don't pick at scabs as they will take longer to heal.

- You may find that you itch like mad and your skin is dry and flaky. Try a rich body lotion, a loofah and oatmeal baths.

- Avoid crash diets and any appetite suppressants or diet drugs for at least 2 weeks after surgery. You need nourishment and lots of H2O, juices and sports drinks in order to heal properly.

- Don't ditch your old wardrobe or go clothes shopping for at least 6 weeks after liposuction, because you will still be shrinking and won't have seen your final result yet.

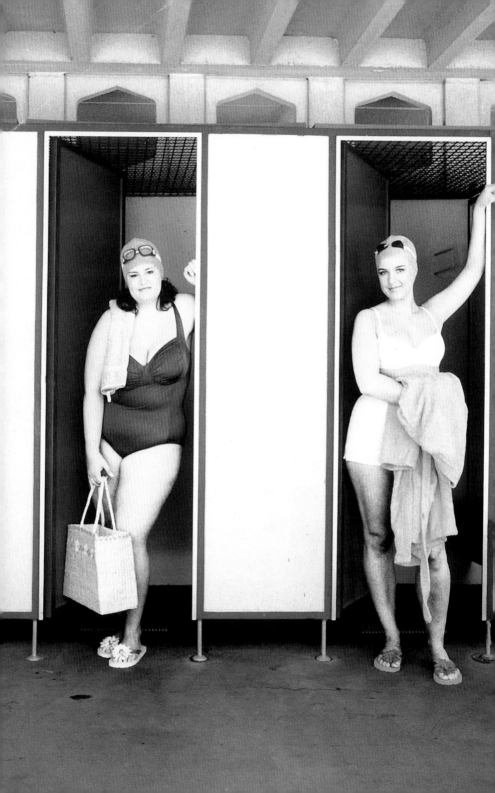

SKINNY SURGERY

The last frontier in figure reshaping is the most radical. If you've done all you can at the gym and the dinner table, there are still several options left to recontour your body back into beautiful form. These should be considered as the last resort, after you have done your part.

If your skin tone is good, you are best served by liposuction. However, if you have an abundance of loose skin on the abdomen or thighs, or have lost a great deal of weight that has left you with a slimmer, but looser body, liposuction won't do the job and may make your ripples look worse. When the degree of skin excess is too severe to be overcome by an exercise regime alone, skin removal in the form of a body lift, is needed. Stand in front of a full length mirror, grab hold of a wad of loose skin and pull up - voila, that's basically what a body lift can do.

If you are severely obese and have several dress sizes to lose to get you healthy, gastric surgery may be suggested, to restrict your food intake so you can lose a lot of weight safely. None of these procedures are quick fixes, and they are not ideal for everybody.

bariatric surgery

Gastrointestinal surgery for obesity helps to restrict food intake by closing off parts of the stomach to make it smaller, or by limiting the absorption of ingested foods.

Since its introduction in 1954, bariatric surgery has become increasingly popular. It is estimated that in 2002, 75,000 people will have the operation in the US alone. Gastrointestinal surgery may be recommended for people who are 7 stone or more over weight and is reserved for those who cannot lose weight by traditional means or who suffer from serious obesity-related health problems. The common measure of obesity is the body mass index, (see page 12). To be eligible for surgery, you have to be 'morbidly obese', or have an index of 40 or above.

The first operation that was widely used for severe obesity was the intestinal bypass, which produced weight loss by causing malabsorption. The concept was that if large amounts of food were eaten, they would be poorly digested or passed along too fast for the body to absorb the calories, but the side effects included a loss of essential nutrients and pain.

The Roux-en-Y: the stomach is separated and a very small pouch is created through stapling or banding to curtail food intake. A Y-shaped section of the small intestine is redirected to the pouch with a narrow opening, bypassing the first and second sections of the intestine to limit food absorption. The procedure requires three days in hospital and a 1 to 3 week recovery. 80% of patients lose at least half their excess weight.

Restrictive surgery also serves to reduce food intake but differs from malabsorptive surgery in that it does not interfere with the digestive process.

Vertical Banded Gastroplasty: the less invasive method that limits food intake by creating a small pouch in the upper stomach. The pouch fills quickly and empties slowly, producing a feeling of fullness. Overeating will result in pain or vomiting and will stretch the pouch. Only half of patients lose at least 50 per cent of their excess weight. This procedure is performed as a day surgery and recovery takes 7-10 days.

LAP-BAND adjustable gastric banding system: a newer method used to limit food intake, whereby a constricting ring is placed completely around the upper end of the stomach just below the junction of the stomach and the oesophagus, creating an hour-glass effect. No cutting or stapling of the stomach is required, the outlet size is adjustable and the band is easily reversible with restoration of normal stomach anatomy after band removal. At present, there are only two devices on the market, and the Lap-Band is only freely available in the US, having been approved for use by the FDA.

These procedures can now be done laparoscopically via a fibre optic tube inserted through small incisions in the abdominal wall. As in other treatments for obesity, the best results are achieved with healthy eating behaviours and regular physical activity. Having the surgery is not a licence to pig out, and compulsive overeaters who don't take charge of their eating disorder can still gain weight after surgery.

body lifts

If sagging and dragging are the problem, a lift may be the only answer. Body lifts are usually performed in tandem with liposuction.

Body lifts are ideal for people who have lost a significant amount of weight and look slimmer overall, but skin stretching with weight gain and shrinking with weight loss has resulted in unattractive laxity. The procedure will remove the redundant skin and is the only technique that can give the patient a pleasing aesthetic look.

The body lift procedure involves the removal of excess skin and fat. The fat is lifted off the muscle and the hanging skin is elevated and tacked into a higher position. Stitches are placed in layers to the deeper structures below and attached to hold the fat and skin securely in place. Ideally, body lifting procedures should be undertaken once you have lost your weight and kept it off long term. Often, multiple stages are required if there are many areas of loose, hanging skin; for example, the lower torso, breasts and arms, and inner thighs and knees.

The body lift procedure has been used in a less advanced form since the 1930s. The modern day procedure has been in use since 1989. The idea behind the body lift is to first use liposuction to contour the underlying fat, smooth it out and then lift the looseness around it. If a patient is having the entire body lift done, they will wear a body girdle postoperatively, for about 2 weeks. The good news for patients is that the incisions are completely hidden in natural skin creases and are not visible in a bathing suit.

Lower Body

The lower body lift was designed to tighten and lift the hips, buttocks and outer thighs all in one stage. It requires an incision around the entire circumference of the abdominal area to remove flabby skin and lift the flank, thigh and buttocks areas. The incision can usually be placed discreetly within standard or high-cut bikini lines. The result of the procedure is a tightened lower back, flank and abdominal skin and removal of cellulite in these areas. The lower body lift is considered among the most invasive of all cosmetic surgery procedures, the recovery is lengthy and scarring is considerable. If inner thighs and saggy knees are the problem, a medial (inner) thigh lift is required. For this an incision is generally placed in the groin area and excess skin is lifted and removed.

Upper Body

Some areas of fat deposits are less forgiving to major fat removal than others, and more often lead to sagging skin; for example, upper arms and inner thighs in women are thinner skinned areas and don't always contract well past the age of 40. For flabby upper arms that don't respond to liposuction alone, an arm lift can be done, that involves a linear incision on the underside of the upper arm from the elbow to the armpit.

fat chances

Imagine if your own fat could be used to create a more appealing physique. Instead of using synthetic materials, fat offers the option of 'like with like' replacement.

When cosmetic surgeons assess your body, they focus on areas that are too full as well as areas that may be fat deficient, such as the buttocks in some women. In order to achieve an ideal curve, a cosmetic surgeon might need to remove fat from one area and add it to a neighbouring one, in order to create an ideal silhouette. Although many women complain of fullness in the hips, some have minor indents that give them a very masculine looking shape. To get a softer, feminine look, some fat may actually need to be added to certain places. The thing to remember about fat, is that you usually don't have enough where you need it and almost always have too much where you don't. It is all about proportions.

Your baby fat may seem to attract the unwanted attention of Great Aunts who can't resist a pinch. But one of the first signs of ageing is the loss of the soft, round, cherubic fullness. As you age, you need all you can get in your face, and it's harder to keep it off your body. The little fat pad under the chin and pouches along the jawline start to expand. By suctioning mini bits of fat, if your skin has good elasticity, it will shrink nicely and give you an improved neck contour. It's a great way to forestall a face-lift, and works well if your chin is weak or if you were just born with a thick, fat neck. It doesn't always work after the mid 40s because skin shrinkage cannot be guaranteed. Women with thicker skin have a better chance of skin contraction.

Filling in the lines

As the natural fat of your face changes shape, hollows start to show up around the eyelids, the middle of the cheeks and around the mouth. An ageing face often appears more square, bottom heavy and angular, as soft tissue slips down from bony structures. It is not uncommon to wonder where your cheekbones have gone and notice that your jawline has lost its sharp, clean angle.

Facial fat doesn't always need to be removed, it often gets redistributed. The century-old technique of fat transplantation has been refined so that fat can be taken from one body area and transplanted as a filler substance to plump up cheeks, chins, furrows and hollows, and fill scars. Putting fullness back into hollows and sunken areas softens the changes associated with ageing. Fat works best as a volume filler for deeper creases and folds, not fine lines. The fat is layered below the skin to create a supportive structure in the face. Donor fat (we've all got some of that) is taken with a small cannula or sterile tube from hips or thighs, processed to remove any blood or serum and then re-injected into the areas to be filled. When done in stages it allows for a gradual improvement over time without a long recovery. Fat transfer is also a wonderful complement to all forms of cosmetic surgery, and new techniques can actually make it last longer. Your fat can be kept frozen for up to a year, which enables additional corrections to be made.

REALITY CHECK: Fat injections do not last forever. For lasting benefits they will have to be repeated.

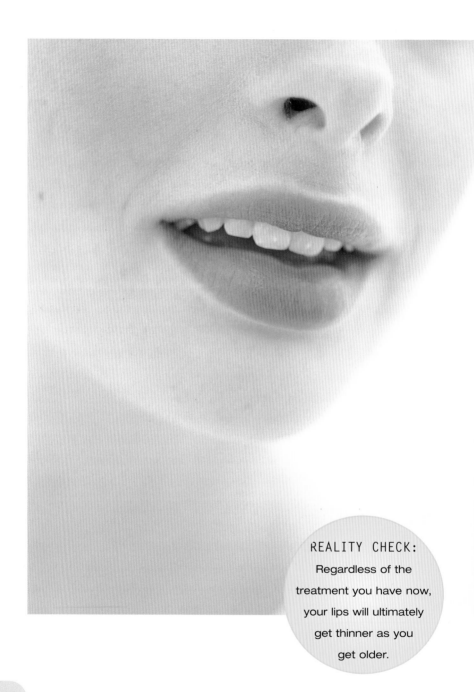

REALITY CHECK:
Regardless of the
treatment you have now,
your lips will ultimately
get thinner as you
get older.

fat lips

Lip augmentation using your own fat is the cosmetic surgeon's treatment of choice. The major advantage is that it is your own so it won't cause an allergic reaction, and most of us have an unlimited supply.

Many features of the ageing face are associated with loss of substance including fat, bone, muscle and connective tissue. Creases, furrows and diminishing lips can be improved by the injection of fat and other filling agents like collagen and hyaluronic acid gel. The benefit of traditional lifting procedures has been contrasted with the less invasive filling approach. Fat can also be used to correct uneven, crooked lips, and even out the top with the bottom or vice versa. The result can be dramatic, fuller and natural, but not if you overdo it. Newly plumped lips have to pass the kiss test. The goal is for lips to look sexy, not scary.

At the beginning of your treatment, your lips should be numbed with a topical anaesthetic to cut down on the 'ouch' factor. Fat can also be put into the lips during a surgical procedure like liposuction or a face-lift, or on its own as a one-time event with a touch-up when you need plumping again. Most surgeons harvest fat with the syringe technique. Because we are constantly using our lips; talking, eating, sipping, yawning, pursing and hailing taxis, even the most brilliantly done fat will only be semi-permanent. Expect to need a few treatments to stay puffy. Lips tend to swell – it may be a few days or a week before they settle down.

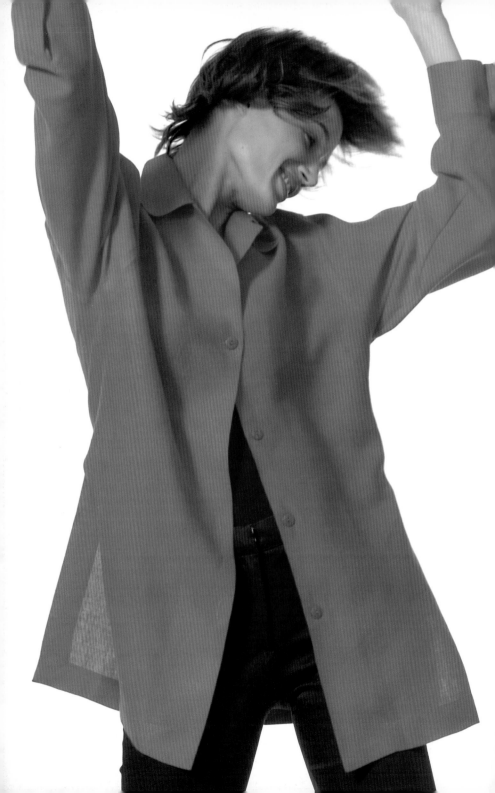

SELF CARE

SELF CARE

Does this make me look fat? If you have to ask, it probably does. Keep it simple. Wear black, or go dark without bold prints, wide stripes or unnecessary trim. To add bright colours, choose those that flatter. Avoid trendy fad colours that are destined to be last year's look before the season ends. Fabrics that move and flow are more slimming than tightly woven or bulky types.

Fit is more important than fashion. Straight-legged trousers are most flattering. Turn-ups shorten the legs. If you're short, skirts should finish just below the knee, or level with the bottom of your calves. Dressing well is about proportion. Short jackets can be deadly if you tend to be bottom-heavy. Try to de-emphasize flaws rather than hide them. Show off your best parts. If you have clothes that you intend to wear when you lose those last 10 pounds, set a time frame. Clothing has a shelf life. Whatever doesn't fit after 6 months, give away. Always try before you buy, or make sure you can return your purchase if the fit isn't great.

You can help your clothes to make you look good by carrying yourself well. Good posture makes your body look better and your clothes drape nicely.

perfect posture

One great way to look 10 years younger is to stand up straight. Having great posture gives you an instant boost in your height and works wonders for your shape.

Keeping your spine in line can improve your physique in a flash. It makes you look taller and slimmer. Good posture can also prevent back problems and the many aches and pains that result from undue stress on joints and muscles. When standing, your head should be over your shoulders, which should not be thrown back. There should be a natural curve to your lower back. Your pelvis should be level and your abdomen should be pulled in. If your pelvis is tipped too far forwards, your stomach will stick out. If it is too far back, the lower back will be too rigid. Straighten your knees, but don't lock them. Finally, your weight should be equally distributed on both legs.

To check the natural curve of your spine, stand with your back, head, shoulders, buttocks and heels flat against the wall. There should be room to slide your fingers between your midback and the wall, but your whole hand shouldn't fit through. If there is room, readjust your stance to reduce the gap. Move your feet forwards so that your back can slide down the wall. Next, rotate your pelvis backwards and tighten your abdominal muscles. Slide back up the wall. The space between your back and the wall should reduce. When walking, take steps of equal length and make sure you have a heel-to-toe gait. Bend your knees and swing your arms naturally at your sides. Before long, as practice becomes habit, you won't have to remind yourself to maintain correct posture. It will become second nature.

Changing shape

Poor posture is tantamount to getting lazy and letting your body go its own way. To adjust your body alignment, train yourself to stop slouching and hunching over by getting your pelvis to tilt correctly. Once you become conscious of your posture, it is important to be aware of it all the time. When you're having a weak moment remember these familiar words: stand up straight, shoulders back, chest out, stomach in.

Your abdominals, lower back muscles, shoulders, gluteals and hamstrings may need strengthening to help you stand up straight comfortably. Exercises that elongate muscles and strengthen joint mobility can add flexibility and strength. Do your exercises in front of a mirror to remind you of your posture. If you sit at a desk all day, stand up to stretch and move around at least every hour, and try sitting in an ergonomic chair.

Yoga – helps improve flexibility, which keeps your muscles supple. It also improves strength endurance, which in turn improves muscle tone and reduces stress. Muscle endurance in the abdomen and spine promotes a strong, healthy back and good posture. It also teaches you how to breathe from your diaphragm. Yoga doesn't punish the body in the way some sports can, and it is perfect for beginners.

Pilates – can dramatically transform the way your body looks, feels and performs by teaching body awareness and flexibility, building strength and promoting graceful movement. It can also help alleviate back pain. Pilates trains several muscle groups at one time in smooth, continuous movements.

know your body type

Every woman has a body type: hourglass v. pear, top heavy or bottom heavy, petite or tall. Make the most of your shape by dressing to accentuate your good parts and hide the bad bits.

A proper fit can cover a multitude of sins. If it isn't pretty, cover it up. If you're busting out of something, throw it away. Start the foundation for your wardrobe with a few key items and build around them:

- Start with a great pair of black fitted trousers. Buy a second pair of black slacks that have a slightly fuller cut.

- Find a short, straight black skirt (above the knee). Add a longer length skirt (below the knee or mid-calf).

- Another must-have: a nice white shirt. Look for some non-bulky basics that you can layer and wear with a variety of items, like turtlenecks and silk sleeveless tops.

- Add a simple solid colour sheath dress; for work it can go under a pretty sweater or jacket then for an evening look, pair it with a shawl.

- Find a basic blazer – in grey, black or navy – that goes with everything and doesn't go out of style.

- Go for suits, but think 'mix 'n' match' – the modern idea of a suit is 2 pieces that work well together but are not necessarily bought as a set.

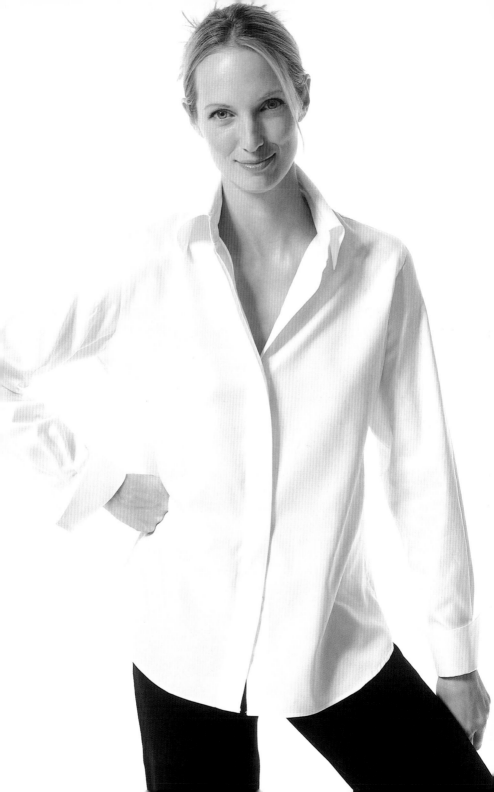

SUMMING IT UP

SUMMING IT UP

It's no secret that women all over the globe are obsessed with their fat cells. According to a recent poll in the US, 71 per cent of women think about their weight at least once a day. For most, dieting is a way of life. The best thing you can do to maintain a healthy perspective is to make peace with your body type. There are 3 danger zones for weight gain in women: at the beginning of your menstrual cycle; after pregnancy; after menopause. The number of fat cells you have is fixed at birth and their distribution is determined by genetics; if you inherited more fat cells on your thighs than on your upper body, you will always have more fat cells there. Gaining or losing weight will increase or decrease the amount of fat in each cell, but it won't alter the number. Coming to grips with the fact that supermodels are born and not made is the first step on the road to taking control of your shape. Starvation diets and liposuction won't give you a 14-inch waist and perfect pins. Setting realistic goals based on what you can and cannot achieve is the key to success.

To lose weight, you have to eat less and exercise more. Despite what you've read, 'Get thin quick' is an oxymoron. Reaching your ideal weight takes time and hard work. Metabolism slows as we age, partially because of decreased activity and muscle mass, and menopause. Dieting further decreases metabolism. However, eating a high-fibre, low-fat diet can reduce weight as well as decrease your chances of developing a disease associated with obesity.

Minimizing cellulite means attacking it with a vengeance. It won't disappear, but with the right exercises, the right equipment and the right diet, you can get it under control. While there are some treatments that can lessen cellulite temporarily, there is no permanent cure.

The good news is that every woman can change her body if she wants to, but it requires a holistic approach. Having high self esteem can help you gain the willpower and commitment to adhere to healthy habits for life. If you need help, don't be afraid to ask a doctor, nutritionist, dietician or personal trainer. Liposuction won't make you thin. It is not a substitute for diet and exercise, and it should be reserved as a last resort or a reward for doing your part. With all of the above you may not end up with a heavenly body, but you'll definitely have a better one.

index

acknowledgments

Special thanks to my gorgeous girl Eden Claire for giving me a reason to write. My great appreciation goes to Alison Cathie and Jane O'Shea for having a vision, and to Lisa Pendreigh and Katie Ginn for making it work.

I also wish to thank the many doctors, surgeons and experts who kindly gave their time and shared their knowledge with me to help with my research. Anita Cela, Sydney Coleman, Dai Davies, Lisa Donofrio, Peter Bela Fodor, Bryan Forley, Laurence Kirwan, Val Lambros, Lyle Leipziger, Z. Paul Lorenc, Timothy Marten, Alan Matarasso, Seth Matarasso, Daniel Morello, Foad Nahai, Malcolm Paul, Nicholas Percival, Gerald Pitman, Barbara Rhea, Rod Rohrich, John Sherman, Howard Sobel, Luis Toledo, Frank Weiser, Patricia Wexler.

picture credits

For more information on achieving a beautiful body visit Wendy Lewis's website at www.wlbeauty.com or email your queries to wlbeauty@aol.com.